Introduction:

You bought the book so thank you, this means you can enter my world of anxiety and general chaos, more than likely you may relate to it.

The goal of this book was not to create a huge novel that you would either get lost in or simply get bored of but to cover some of my life, the issues I have faced and in turn hopefully help you.

They do say less is more and I hope that will shine through in this short book, the aim of which, is to show you that you are not alone and what you are experiencing may also be the issues of so many other people including myself.

It took me some time to realise it but one thing I have now learned is that I am not alone and neither are you.

Let's walk together through this book and by the end of it you may have related to many of my issues.

You may well be able use this book to look back at when things get too much for you and remind yourself of what you have read and perhaps how to cope with it.

CONTENTS

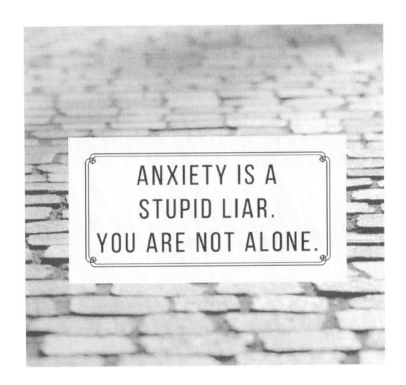

ANXIETY IS A
STUPID LIAR.
YOU ARE NOT ALONE.

Who is the Anxiety bloke?

My name is Bradley Allan, I have issues, lots of bloody issues.

I am a married 39-year-old father of 3.

I am not a writer, in fact I flunked English at school and this is the first thing I've ever put effort into when it comes to writing.
The thought of writing down my feelings and issues is overwhelming but at the same time it's already making me feel like I have a sense of purpose.

For many years I had no idea or understanding why I acted and felt like I did and was not just scared of how I acted and felt but also embarrassed, speaking up was just not an option and I felt very much alone.

Over the years I have read many books on anxiety and mental health, but very few actually made me feel like I understood what the writer was really saying and I felt like I just couldn't relate to them, in reality they are mostly the same text book approach that I've read over and over where I give up reading and the book is thrown with the rest of my failed purchases.

I find it very frustrating that someone can write a book on Anxiety because they have studied it but never experienced or felt it.

I have attended multiple counselling sessions, listened to dozens of self-help apps on my phone, viewed dozens of hypnoses on YouTube yet I am still the same person and often living my daily nightmare.

I have tried CBT (Cognitive Behavioural Therapy) which did help but like most things my head and train of thought soon over ruled it, perhaps if I had tried it before I got to the level of Anxiety I have now it may have worked better for me, if it works for you great but we are all different when it comes to coping and conquering.

I do believe CBT has its place and I will cover how it went for me and how I tweaked what I learned to help me personally.

I have searched for books and articles for many years to give me that cure or at least where I could relate to what I was reading but it was the same text book type stories and the same ways on how we should cope, that would be great if we were Robots and all made the same but we are not.

When I told my best mate I was writing a book he laughed and said you can barely write a Facebook post that makes sense never mind a book about Anxiety.

Virtually every book I have read on Anxiety is either complicated and fries my head or is just plain damn boring…. that is what fuelled this book in the first place.

Over the years many people have asked me what can I have to worry about and why would I suffer anxiety, there is no reason, I just have it. Simple

I look and act just like most guys or at least I try and act like most guys.
Front the outside I am pretty powerfully built guy having enjoyed lifting weight for quite a few years, I have lots of tattoos and I can come across as a bit of a character but I can also be very weak and crippled with issues when anxiety grips hold of me and takes control.

People often say how confident I come across and when anxiety isn't present in my head I actually can be a pretty confident person in the right situation.

It took me a long time to understand my anxiety and just how far it would push me, not many people realise but anxiety is a medical condition and you do need to treat and understand it just like any other illness, just *how* you do that varies from person to person but I hope this book helps even a little bit towards that.

Anxiety is not a sign of weakness, as many people think and can actually be a sign of strength.
More often people with anxiety will soldier on for months or many years before seeking treatment, I know I certainly did and for such a long time was almost oblivious to just how crazy my life had become.

Google has millions of articles on Anxiety but they seldom helped me, I like real-world talk and real-world scenarios and that is the aim of this book.

The biggest challenge for many of us is admitting there is something not quite right with us, for many of us it's the fear of being judged or even embarrassed.

I thought about writing this book for quite a few years but often decided against it because I was worried what others would think, would I be judged, would I be laughed at, the thought of people knowing my inner truths and flaws was quite scary but only now do I realise what I once thought were flaws are far more common than most us realise and I have learned is no one is perfect.

I spent many years thinking no one understood and that I was alone but in reality, that was miles from the truth and people do understand, it was me who was holding back from giving them the chance to understand.
People may not understand just how bad anxiety makes you feel and just how low it can drag you down but that's fine, you don't need them to understand it at that level, the most important person to understand is YOU.

I have lots of stories and over the last 20+ years nearly all of them have stuck with me and left me with the memories I carry every single day, some great and some not so great.

I am constantly exhausted from worrying about every little detail and when my next anxiety attack will be.

I am just a normal looking bloke who on the outside looks like most other guys, by day I work in a pretty decent job and by night when not running about after my loveable kids (I best say that) I can be found at the gym acting and looking like a stereotypical tattooed meathead, that's of course if I can walk through the bloody gym door without having a meltdown or sitting in my car debating just going home again.

This book is to show you that you're not alone.
I want to be open and honest about the many times where I felt like I just couldn't go on, felt like I was alone and no one understood.

There are many people who have also suffered because of my anxiety and I failed to recognise it.

Anxiety will grab hold of you so bad that nothing or nobody else matters and loved ones and friends will be pushed away or treated unfairly and we often don't even realise we are doing it.

I don't know what drives me more to write this book, the fact of being able to write down my past and current issues or the fact I may well be helping you understand and relate to what I am saying.

There is also a part of me is using this book to let my friends, family and loved ones know that I now recognise my illness has made me treat them unfairly but I am now working on it and fighting back against anxiety, just like you can.

People often say to me that it's all in my head, do they honestly think I want to feel how I do?

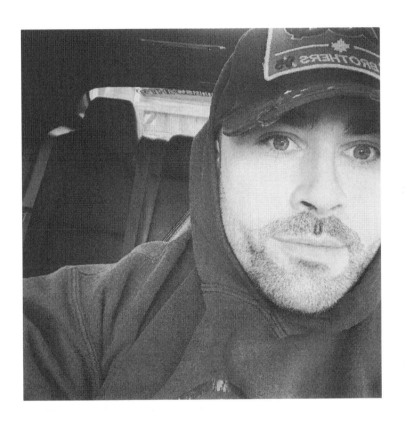

Bradley Feb 2019

CHAPTER ONE

Lovable Rouge

Lovable rouge, that's the name given to me over the years by friends, family and those who have come in and out of my life, but over the years that has been changed thanks to my behaviour and actions.

I know I've led a colourful life, it's had some crazy ups and downs with many obstacles, but we only get one shot at life and it's very much what we make it.

In my younger years I was no angel, I often skipped school, had some run ins with the law and on many occasions was told by my parents and people of authority that I needed to sort myself out.
There was a period of around 5 years where I drastically went off the rails and my life seemed to be heading nowhere good and I just didn't know why or how to stop it.

From the outside I am that stereotypical lucky guy, nice family life, nice cars, great job, nice and healthy and always working out in the gym or doing sports, sounds bloody great, doesn't it?

"He can't have problems" most people would say and pass comments saying my life looks great, I wish I had some of what he has, the nice cars, the nice house but in reality, all of the above was a massive front and couldn't be further from the truth, my life was not great and I was far from perfect.

Trust me a flashy life or existence means jack shit when you're breaking bit by bit from the inside.

Anxiety can not only ruin the life of the person that it has hold of but also their loved ones and you can't see or understand why.

If you ask my ex-wife or family if I am a nice guy, you'll certainly not think that I am after a few minutes.
I have spent many years of accusing my ex-wife of not understanding and lashing out at her verbally in my frustration, in fact I have lashed out at many people over the years for no reason other than it was the only reaction I had when I felt like how I did and on many occasions then trying to justify to myself that it was okay to act how I just did, most times it was far from okay.
I had been unreasonable and not in control of myself and that, I now understand.

When your head is so consumed with worry it makes it very difficult to control our reactions and how we speak to and deal with other people, at that point in time our head tells us that no one else matters but us.

Only now when I look back do I understand the crazy amount of times where I've acted like nothing short of an absolute wanker and those around me didn't deserve to be on the brunt of how I have felt.

Setting the scene

Let's set the scene for you as I feel it's important, I am not a writer, I am certainly not a mental health worker and I am sure as hell no expert when it comes to mental health. Anxiety is a condition I have suffered with for a long time and it is something I am still trying to understand but I have become somewhat better and my understanding of which, continues to improve.

One thing I am, is a realist and if only I had spoken up years ago and faced reality and taken action then, I guess I wouldn't be here writing this or certainly not in the mess I am in.

I have issues, lots of issues, you might have issues too and one thing I've recently learned is that nor you or I are alone when it comes to this rollercoaster that we are on.

I'm not rare or special and I will not sugar coat my life past nor present, my sole reason for writing this book is to speak about the things that have happened almost daily for the last 20 years.

I dare say when I read them back I will understand that 99% of it was bullshit and that I really shouldn't have let it consume me but it did and it broke me, hopefully it makes you think and understand that what you feel shouldn't consume you.

I hope you read this and can perhaps relate some of it to your world or gain an understanding of how someone around you may be feeling.

This book will shock you but hopefully allow you to walk my journey with me and make sense to many times or situations you may also have suffered.

On paper, I look like any other normal happy guy and over the years people have become aware of my anxiety and often pass comments saying that I can't have anxiety and that alone has in many situations, made how I've felt and acted 100 times worse.

I genuinely don't think I can't handle one more person telling me it's all in my head and just to ignore it, you try ignoring something that is consuming every thought and feeling at that moment in time.

Anxiety does not pick who it latches itself to and in many cases most of us don't know we even suffer it until it's already taken control of our lives and mental state.

**People will say they understand…
We will say they don't.**

**People will say to just snap out of it…
We won't**

**People will tell us that it's no big deal…
It's a huge deal.**

But I am telling you one important thing and something that you and I need to remember and that's the fact we are not alone, we don't need everyone to understand how we feeling or the exact level of our issues, if they understand then great if they don't then don't waste time letting their lack of understanding fuel negative thoughts.

We are more powerful than we will realise, there will be good days where we can kick anxiety in the face and there will be bad days when we cannot, one phrase that I have taught myself and I will most likely use it throughout this book is "Every day can be a progress day"

It's quite ironic that I am writing this book because other than my best mate, no one knows I am writing this and even my mate thinks I will run out of things to think or say, that's quite ironic because I have a million things I want to say and share.

I have a million things in my head that can and will consume me if I let them.

I have always been ambitious when it comes to things like my career and like to push myself at everything I do in life and this book has been something I have wanted to write for quite a few years, if even one person relates to how I feel and act and it is even a tiny bit of help for them then it's all been worthwhile.

I would say I am a deep person and I always play my cards close to my chest, too close in fact.

Being such a deep person and not one to speak much or share my feelings has had a huge impact on how I have grown into the person I am today, I am very much a closed book or at least I was until now.

They do say sometimes you need to hit rock bottom before you can start your fight to be a better, healthier and certainly a more manageable person so I guess this is my rock bottom, this is my new start and my fight to beat my issues and perhaps help you beat yours.

Remember:

YOU
MATTER.

CHAPTER TWO

Growing up

I am quite lucky that I grew up in an era where things like social media, games consoles and computers didn't really exist, our house TV worked on 50 pence coins so if there was no money, there was no TV to watch.

I grew up in pretty rough and ready but great council estate in Aberdeen, our house was on the 18th floor of a high rise flat, an absolute bitch for me because from a very young age I was scared of going in the flat lift so it meant climbing 18 floors of stairs to get to my house, on many occasions I would get to the bottom to have to go all the way back up again, to this day I am still scared of lifts and refuse to set foot in one.

"Lifts bloody terrify me"

Lifts to this day still bloody terrify me, I have on many occasions tried to get over this fear and within seconds of setting foot in one I start to sweat and my heart is racing, I will have thoughts in my head about the lift cables snapping or the lifting getting stuck or being stuck and there is no oxygen and I suffocate, all crazy thoughts but at that moment in time they will feel very much real, it's not just lifts, I hate all confined spaces and the thought of being stuck in any small space will put my anxiety through the roof.

Back to growing up, the area I stayed although badged and often spoken about as being rough was actually a friendly place back then and everyone knew everyone, growing up in the 80s was a great time, things were just so much bloody easier.

I come from a working class family and growing up my father worked as a welder in a ship yard and Mum did various jobs from cleaner to being a home help for old age pensioners, money was always tight and I was taught and respected the value of money from a very early age, if I wanted to have fun or experience things then it meant getting my ass outside with friends and making the best of things that cost absolutely nothing.

I would spend my days with friends climbing virtually everything we could or being chased for being cheeky little shits was a daily occurrence.

There was no shite like Facebook where someone could mail your mum and dad and say what you had been up to, if they wanted to tell your folks they had to visit your house and that seldom happened.

There was no snapchat or phones lurking to film what you were doing, there was no Instagram to show random people what you were doing just to get some likes, god it was a great time to be alive

There was no heroin addicts or junkies walking the streets back then and things like scum bag paedophiles and nonces were an unknown, from a very young age you could go

play on the streets and parks with your mates with no care about any of the above, your only care was when your Mum came looking for you to get your ass home.
The fact there were no mobile phones for your mum to phone you to come home, in fact we didn't even have a house phone so it was a common occurrence to hear my mum's voice screaming from afar to get my arse home.

Life was good as a kid, it was tough but looking back I had no real worries.

Looking back my only real worry I can remember is when I was around 10 I woke one night to find my mum in tears to hear that my grandma had died, I didn't really understand much other than everyone was upset and that I kept hearing them say that my grandad would have to come with live with us, staying in the flat meant this just wasn't possible so we would have to move house.
I didn't understand why we had to move but we did and it happened extremely quickly.

Moving house

At the age of 10 I moved away to another area of Aberdeen and I instantly lost all my friends which broke my heart for days on end, I felt like running away and I went from being a care free young lad to an emotional wreck, the thought of losing my friends terrified me, to make things worse I was told that I was also moving schools as it just wasn't possible to keep going to the same school, they were only 3 miles apart but back then even a bus pass was a luxury and my mum had a part time job so couldn't take me to my old school.

It was a lot to take in and even as a 10-year-old it was tough on my head and still to this day I remember it like it was yesterday.

The house move happened scarily fast and a few weeks passed and my first day at my new school had arrived, only now when I look back do I realise this is where I became a nervous and anxious person.

That morning I was literally dragged to school kicking and screaming, at one point as we reached the school gates I broke free of my mum's grip and ran away from her, it took her nearly 2 hours to calm me down and get me to go in to the school.

29 years later I still remember that morning like it was yesterday, as I entered the class the teacher stopped what she was doing to greet me and asked me to take a seat, she then went on to introduce me to the entire class, I still remember every kid looking and staring at me.

I was convinced they had seen me run away earlier that morning and that they were all speaking about and laughing at me, the whole day I just wanted to get home and back into my room, it was like that most days and I took a long time to build up the confidence to speak to the other kids in the class.

It's only all these years later that I realise how much those changes at a young age had affected me, since that day I've struggled with change and often worry about what breaking my routine will do or how it will make me feel.

I now hated school, it took me months to build a circle of friends and even then I always felt on edge, I used to say to my mum I didn't feel well, when she asked me what was wrong I would always say I didn't know, that was common and for many years I had those feelings and had days off school.

Things got better when moving up to secondary school and I had a small circle of friends, I was often in trouble and the teachers called me a trouble maker on many occasions, I don't believe I was, I was just always so bloody confused and craving understanding.

I would often get invited to sports clubs or out of school activities, but I never went and always felt too nervous and on many occasions the thought of it scared me, back then I had no idea why other than it was easier to not go and just go walking about the streets with my mates instead.

I was a bit of a class clown at times who got the odd detention and punishment, but I stuck it out and my grades were semi decent.

I actually liked secondary school and I had a great close circle of friends many of whom I am still friends 20 years later, at school I was by no means an angel and my friends and I would often spend our time climbing the school roofs or causing some sort of mischief but that's just what kids do, I was a colourful teenager behaviour wise that's for sure.

Leaving school should have been a great time and I couldn't wait to join the working world.

I had been looking for jobs and I knew it had to be something hands on where I could get my hands dirty, I liked messing about in my older brothers' car so working in a garage was where all my applications were being sent.

I received some news that I secured an apprenticeship at a local car garage which was exactly what I wanted and would be starting the week after leaving school.

Thinking back this is where life got real and I didn't realise in the next few years I was about to go from a boy to a man and rapidly.

Joining the real world

Something you don't quite realise as a naive 16-year-old is that when you enter the working world and become an adult is that you now have responsibilities and consequences for your actions are much severe.

As an adult you're not only now part of the bigger world but you're exposed to so much more and I truly believe this is where my anxiety started to creep out and grab hold of me.

I couldn't just take days off work like I did at school and everyone seemed to look at what I did so much more than they did when I was a kid.

When I was at school, I said I couldn't wait to leave and every adult used to tell me they wished they were back at school, that was very much true.
School was such an easier life with no responsibilities other than get good grades and there was no real scrutiny like we get as adults.

My first job and step into the working world

My first day at my new job and stepping into the working world soon arrived and the first few months were great, and the new start nerves soon passed.
Everyone seemed so nice and helpful and although I didn't realise at the time the transition from a naive school boy into an adult was almost overnight when I entered the real world and stepped away from my comfort zone.

I was enjoying getting up each day to put a boiler suit on and being "one of the boys" at work.

Being 16 is an age where we are very naïve and impressionable so as an apprentice, I get sucked into the older boy's stories that they'd tell and the bravado they had of being better than the guy sitting next to them.

Every day I would listen to the guys as they had a new story about the shit they had done or were going to do, this ranged from girls they had slept with to the drugs they had taken, the sort of stuff as a 16 year old you just sit and listen to and suck it all it but you would never tell your parents.

It turned out after a few months that my boss was what I can only describe as a modern-day Hitler and started to take a dislike to me or just plain liked to bully young kids.

I was 16 and this guy was about 50, his day consisted of picking faults at every piece of work I did and pretty much bullying me non-stop.

This guy would come up behind me and nip my ears or slap me on the back of the head just for a laugh, if I said anything, I just got it ten times worse.
This asshole's bullying killed my confidence and I dreaded work every single day, I was scared to be around the guy but in my head I had kicked the shit out of him a million times.

Every day he would pick at me and looking back this is where I started to suffer my first bouts of anxiety, it got to the point I was scared to go to work and the night before work I would sit in my room pancaking and feeling all sorts of emotions, only now do I realise that what I was suffering was anxiety thanks that piece of shit who honestly made me feel unworthy in the work place .
Work was a place with everything going on, at home I really hoped would be a safe place; an environment where I could feel happy.

My dad is a pretty switched on guy.
I was starting to take days off work as I felt almost ill at the thought of going each day and he soon noticed it.
He asked what the issue was and I told him how my boss was towards me and the sort of things he would do.

My dad being the guy he is said "look it's not a problem let's just go have a chat with your boss and see what this guy is saying".

My dad is a strong character, he doesn't suffer fools easily and back then he wasn't the type to be intimidated unlike me.

The next day as he drove me to work, I felt physically sick, what if my boss said I was lying, what if my boss said I was fired, and the thoughts in my head were all over the place I couldn't control them. Anxiety has that effect, almost similar to other mental illnesses.

To say I was a nervous wreck would've been an understatement, what happened next was something that I'll never forget. Dad asked him how I was getting on and my boss said "yes, Bradley is doing great, he is a nice kid and a right good worker".

At this point my dad then asked him why he felt the need to pick on a 16 year old boy and to "stop speaking fucking shite" and "pick on someone his own size", at that point my boss then verbally attacked my dad and told him to get the fuck out of his garage before he called the police..
My dad told me to pop back to the car, I ran back and locked the doors.
I could see my dad arguing and my boss standing there looking scared, it felt great.
My Dad grabbed my toolbox and walked back to the car with not a care in the world.
I will never know what was said to my Boss that day by my dad but damn it felt great to see him put my Boss where he belonged, the guy was an asshole.
My Dad was my hero that day.
He simply got back in the car and said "Son, I think we need to find you a new job, there is no time in life for bullies".
I just sat there all smug and proud of my dad and of course I couldn't wait to tell my mates what had just happened at work.

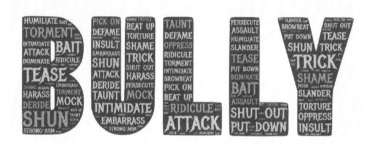

No one likes a Bully in life

On the Job hunt

The next day I contacted nearly every garage in the local area to see if any jobs could be had, a few weeks went past and I was offered another job with a local main dealer who sold Vauxhalls, a garage 10 times the size of the last place I worked and it had dozens more staff, I was excited but I was also terrified.

The garage was around a 40-minute drive from my house but dad had agreed to drop and collect me each day until I passed my driving test which meant I didn't need to worry about getting there.

First day and a new start

My first day arrived and I just couldn't drag myself into the car to head to the garage, my mum was asking me what was wrong but I didn't know, I was pouring with sweat and felt physically sick, my dad eventually got me in the car and off we went, I'll never forget how nervous I was that day.
I was like a block of ice, scared to move or say anything, this was an anxiety attack, back then I didn't know what it was but all these years later, I now do.

As the weeks and months went past it was a great place to work and everyone was great, I was learning new skills and my new boss was a good guy, he was strict and a real tough character, but he wasn't a bully unlike the last asshole that I had worked for previously.

The guys I worked with soon became friends and the job was great, the feelings of worry that I had previously experienced had totally vanished and I loved going to work.

It was tough to begin with, having to learn so many new things and often being pushed to get things done in a certain time or having my new boss watch over me but they were pretty good at spotting when I was struggling and often leant a hand.

A couple of years passed at the job with no issues and I was a happy go lucky lad, I could be a cheeky shite at times but the guys at work gave as good back and there was often some workplace banter and tricks played on each other.

It was common to almost need eyes in the back of your head wondering what one of the other guys was going to try and do to you, always trying to outdo each other.

"I won't go into the day I had my balls greased"

I won't go into the day I had my balls greased by the older lads, all in fun and I took it well.

Try that in today's politically correct society and the youth of today would be running to their boss to report harassment in hope of a big fat claim.

I have many fond memories of my time at that place and the things that went on and the many skills that I had learned.

One valuable thing I learned is never superglue your bosses' juice cap to his bottle, the glue often won't dry and you end up gluing the 6ft5' tank of a man's Glaswegian lips.

I think I covered 5k that day being chased around the garage by that absolute unit of a guy, all in fun once he calmed down, a brilliant memory.

Time passed and I had now passed my driving test and had bought my own first car.

The other guys I worked with would often help me work on my car and it became my pride and joy, the perks of free bits also meant I managed to turn my few hundred quid pile of shit into a pretty tidy motor.

Passing a driving test is every teenagers dream but for me this was about to turn into a living nightmare.

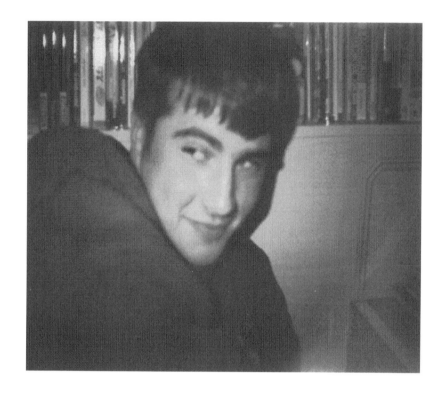

Picture: 18 Years old and oblivious to what was about to happen next

CHAPTER THREE

The Outsider

I was now 18 and my parents dropped the bombshell they had decided that they wanted to move to the countryside to get away from the noise and stress of the city centre life.

They picked a remote location some 30 miles from Aberdeen, all my friends were in Aberdeen so this meant during the week I was isolated and had no friends, after work I would be stuck in the house.
I couldn't cope with being stuck in the house and fond out there was a small town some 10 miles away with people my age.

They had what they called a circuit where the younger lot drove about in their cars, pretty much going around in circles.

I decided to drive up one night and see what was going on and sure enough there were lots of cars and girls going about.

This became a regular thing and it wasn't long before my car was getting a fair bit of attention form the locals, working in a garage I had the time and equipment to make my car look a bit different and modify how it looked, my car was my pride and joy.

The town was a bloody strange place where everyone knew everyone and they didn't like outsiders, it was like going back in time compared to the large town I had been brought up in.

One night I decided to head into the local town for a drive about and picked up one of the local girls that I had been speaking to for a few weeks, we drove about just chatting away and listening to my dire taste in music.

We drove about like everyone else, going around in circles, it was the thing to do and although these days I would rather watch paint dry it was the done thing as spotty teenager.

That evening we had been driving about for around 30 minutes when I spotted a large group of guys pointing at me in an aggressive way, I asked the girl who they were and she said "oh. just ignore them, they don't like strangers in their town", I was a pretty cocky teen back then and in my head I wasn't intimated but thinking back I was pretty anxious at what might happen, but I did think at the time about my dad's words over the years, I decide to not let these bullies chase me away so the girl and I went for some food and a drive.

An hour later as I drove back into the town I was met with the same group of guys stood at the road side, one suddenly jumped onto the road and into the path of my car, he had kicked the side of my car, I lost control and had ending up pinning the young lad against a wall with my car…in a split second my world had just crumbled.

I ran out of the car to see the young guys legs being crushed by my car against a solid granite wall, it seemed like hours, but moments later the police and ambulance arrived, and the guy was freed and taken to hospital.

I was arrested by the police and placed in a holding cell in the local police station, I was 19 and although I had the odd silly dealing with the police as a kid, I had never been placed in handcuffs and thrown into a jail cell.

By now I wasn't having an anxiety attack, I had skipped that and I was having what I now know was a full-blown panic attack, I couldn't breathe and the size of the cell just kept feeling smaller and smaller, I was banging on the door but no one would come, I was trapped in a room and situation that I had no escape from.

I lay down on an old grey blanket and somehow managed to nod off, I woke up abruptly as the door swung open to be met with two men dressed in suits... "Bradley we are CID from Peterhead, we need you to come with us please", my heart sank...

"Have I killed that I guy?" I asked

"Can I call my dad" I said

No answer was given apart from just come with us please. The handcuffs went back on, I was led outside and into the back of an unmarked car, we then drove to Peterhead police station where I was checked in and they explained an interview would be carried out. They had to do their job and ask questions.

The only time I've ever seen this was on TV, I asked for my one phone call and they just laughed and threw me back in a cell.

A few hours went past and the cell door opens, I tell them that I can't breathe and I feel sick, they ignore what I say and lead me to a tiny room with 4 seats, a desk and a tape recorder.

The thoughts in my head were all over the place, I couldn't focus and there was a fear of impending doom going around and around in my head.

Inside the room they explained that the interview would be recorded, and they caution me just like you see on TV. They ask me to tell them exactly what happened, I tell them exactly how it was, that the group of guys were on the road and one of them kicked my car and that I lost control, "it happened so quickly" I said.

There were lots of pauses and it was like they were waiting for me to say something that at the time, I knew would land me in some serious shit so I just said as little as I could. One of the officers started talking to me, looking straight at me like I was some youth murderer.

"Is that your final statement Bradley? Please think carefully before saying yes or no"

I simply nodded and said "yes it is".
"Ok Bradley" the officer says, "I would like to advise you that on today's date you did in fact intentionally run over a person ***** ***** with full intent to cause harm and serious injury therefore at this date and time you are being charged with attempted murder, you do not have to say anything but anything do say may be given or used in evidence". I was stunned. I just sat there.

"Do you have anything to say?"

Eventually I blurted out.. "No I don't."

I was released on bail pending a trial, this seemed to drag on for ever and as the months went passed my worry about what was going to happen got worse and worse, eventually my day in court arrived some 10 months later.

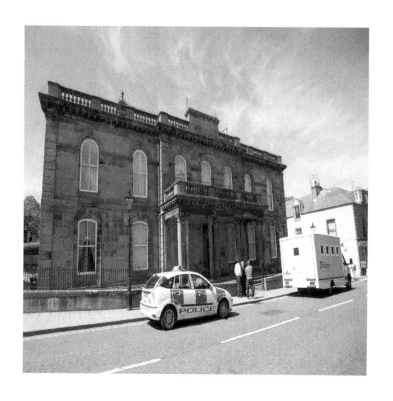

Banff Sheriff Court, Aberdeenshire

Day of the Trial

My day at court finally arrived which was held at Banff sheriff court in Aberdeenshire, meeting with my solicitor that morning we chatted about my options and he told me the PF (Procurator Fiscal) said if I plead guilty to a lesser charge of serious assault or dangerous driving it would all be dealt with today and I could put it behind me, looking back the whole thing was a joke and I still believe that the court system is corrupt and deals are made behind closed doors based on who you are.

My solicitor who was supposed to be the best and advised me to take the deal as there were several people saying I had ran the guy over on purpose and were prepared to stand as witnesses, he advised me to just get it over with to keep me out of jail.

Looking back, he wasn't intrusted in taking it to full trial and it's now clear he just wanted to move on to his next case and make a fast buck for very little hassle.

I was advised to agree to the dangerous driving option which I did, we were called up into the court room and I confirmed my name, my solicitor read out my plea and the judge, after a few minutes of speaking gave up his sentence to me.... 5-year driving ban and £2500 fine.

The whole process took less than an hour and I was on my way home.

Looking back, it's only now do I realise that I had just obtained a criminal record that would sit with me for the rest of my life when I should have fought against the charge and took my chances but back then I wasn't even bothered, I just wanted out of that court and to put that insane part of my life behind me.

The next day I went back to work as usual and within minutes I was called into my boss's office, "Bradley we need to let you go" he said, he then went on to explain that a driving licence was essential for my job and insurance purposes, I didn't know what to say or do so I just said I understood.

I called my dad to explain and he came and collected me, and that was the end of that career, at the time I was devastated as I loved that job.

CHAPTER FOUR

Falling into a Rut

After being let go from the garage I went through a few years of dead end jobs that were leading to nowhere, I would look for any excuse as to why I didn't like the job or any excuse to not turn up.

I reckon in a period of around 5 years I must have had around 30+ jobs, most of which last weeks or months at most.

Every day waking up was like someone had sucked the life from me, I had no desire to do anything other than get past the day and on to the next. I would stay in bed all day and go out at night, there was no routine.
I don't know where my head was at and I don't really have a valid excuse, all I know is that no matter what I did I always failed and ended up back where I started.

I done many dodgy deals back in the day to make a few quid, many of which were illegal but if it made me money then I would turn my hand to it, I would go through periods where I had no money for weeks on end or a sudden influx where I had so much of it that I didn't know what to do with it, I would need a book in itself to speak about the sort of shit I got up to back then, some good and some not so good.

I had various stints working part time as a doorman at nights which was quite ironic as I didn't like being around people that I didn't know but it was a job and one I was surprisingly good at, back then you didn't need to pass any criminal record checks and the jobs were mostly secured through recommendations from other doorman who knew you could handle yourself and knew you would have their back if shit went wrong.

The doorman community back then in Aberdeen was a pretty small circle of guys who all knew each other and clubs had far less trouble than they do now, known idiots were kept from getting in and anyone kicking off inside would be dealt with quickly and it would be made sure they knew not to take the piss again, our sole aim as doormen was to keep people safe and keep the not so friendly under control.

Many of the guys I worked with were top blokes and the rumours of doorman being bullies or trouble makers back then were seldom true, you try having some junkie pull a needle on you or a pissed guy smash a bottle over your head and see how you react to the situation.

Being a doorman for about 10 hours a week was never going to make me financially okay or lead to anything good and I was spending everything I made in the casino at the end of each shift, so it was a pointless effort.
Back then I had no drive and my only desire was to get through each day in the hope the next day would be better and some amazing job would land on my lap and I would be able to leave that pub doorway and stop dealing with the same pished idiots every night.

On many occasions I would be wrestling about the floor with group of people and being paid pennies for it.

Being a doorman was such a public facing job and although I struggled to walk into a pub on my own or sober I could easily stand on a door, not bat an eye lid and do a good job, it was one of the few jobs where I felt in control and anxiety didn't really bother me when I was standing on that door.

Looking back anxiety played a huge part my private life and as soon as I finished a shift or was back home things started to escalate, back then no one had any idea just how I was behind closed doors and just how much power my head had over me.

I was leading two lives, the confident doorman at night and the stay at home anxious guy by day.

I was also now a father, this should have been the wakeup call I needed but my son's mother soon got fed up and we parted ways.

I had no desire to do things or better myself and I wasn't seeing my son, I generally wasn't a very nice person and it was easier to lock myself in the house most days, the thought of going out to get a real job or fixing my life just wasn't an option.

You hear about people losing faith in others but I had lost faith in myself and I didn't know how to snap out of it.

CHAPTER FIVE

Pulling myself together

Thankfully I met a new partner and although she could see I had some issues she was prepared to give me a chance and we moved in to together.

I managed to secure myself a new job within the Oil Industry, it was a trainee position starting at the bottom and the money was poor but at the end of the day it was a job and a reason to get up each day.

I didn't even have to attend an interview, a local agency called me and asked if I was looking for work and before I knew it was starting the following Monday.

The minute I hung up the phone I was overcome with many mixed emotions, excited but also nervous, what if someone asked where I had worked the last few years, what if someone knew about my past or what if someone didn't like me, what would I do, the thoughts in my head were all over the place, this went on for days until the Monday finally arrived and my dad arrived to pick me up, I had thought of probably a dozen reasons why I shouldn't go but it was too late, I was in the car and heading for my new job….absolutely terrified.
When we arrived I checked in at reception and waited for what seemed like a decade but in reality it was a matter of

minutes before a guy a appeared and took me through to the workshop where I was going to be working, walking to the workshop we had to pass a load of people and I could feel my heart racing and I was aware that I was avoiding making eye contact with any of them.

I still remember that day like it was yesterday and just how aware I was of how I was acting and thinking, worrying all day that something bad was going to happen. It never did. A few weeks passed and the job had given me a sense of purpose again and although there were many occasions where I felt like I couldn't turn up or wasn't able to face anyone I fought through it and kept pushing forward. I guess I wanted to prove to myself I could do it and show others I could too.

The job progressed to me working away from home and this meant travelling offshore on the oil rigs or overseas, this posed a whole new level of anxiety where I was away from loved ones and now having thoughts like never before.

What if something happened to me while I was away, I was having thoughts in my head and these were new to me. I had never thought about dying before and these thoughts were now added to my list of worries and attacks that I would have.

There were occasions where they got so bad that I would make an excuse so I had to travel home early which put my job at risk. I was obsessed with the thought of dying and leaving my loved ones behind, these attacks always led on to more and more attacks and although it put huge strain on my job I had to battle through them, I would speak to doctors when I was away and they would just tell me it was normal and not to worry, worrying was something I had become an expert at.

I was told what I had was Thanatophobia which is the technical term for worrying about death but in my head these technical terms and meanings meant nothing to me nor did I care, all I cared about was not feeling like I did and things just seemed to get worse and worse.
If I wasn't worried about dying, I was worried about what people thought about me at work, I dare say I became a very paranoid person.

Over the next 13 years I phased out working part time as a doorman and went on to grow my career and learn many new skills whilst battling anxiety and the many scenarios it would throw at me.
There have been good days, many bad ones and looking back I guess they inspired me to write this book in the first place.

I know how alone it can be and how bloody scary it can become when everyone just wants you to appear okay and be "normal".

The false smiles, the fake saying you're ok and the putting on an act for places like work or events.

At times it can all seem too much but trust me it does and will get better, I tell myself that most days and it's common for me to stop and remember where I once was.

One thing I have learned is to be upfront with people if you can and more so in your working life, if you're less worried about what people think or not trying to hide your issues then you're less likely to worry and it will minimise the amount of attacks.

In many ways I was now using my passion for my career to keep my head and thoughts busy and in turn minimise overthinking as much as I could, I strongly believe keeping the head active keeps anxiety at bay.

I have since gone on to become self-employed and set up several businesses, some failed and some to this day are a success, I often tell myself that I am juggling two jobs, one being my career and the other my Anxiety.

CHAPTER SIX

The scary and irrational side of anxiety

There is absolutely no doubt that my anxiety on many occasions has made me a very irrational and almost aggressive person.

Over the years this illness has made me have some crazy thoughts, these kinds of thoughts consume you and in turn leave you almost angry that you have been thinking them. This bloody illness will turn even the simplest of things into the biggest deal in the world and as much as people may say it's no big deal it will be a huge one to us.

Looking back and now, understanding myself better than ever I can't believe just how easily I can become disappointed in even the tiniest of things.

It took me a long time to understand that anxiety will trigger a stress response in the body and in turn leave me feeling stressed at so many things that any normal person would be able to just brush off.

Couple all of this together and you then have a very much out of control head that can't think straight and allows us to be wide open to thinking irrationally.

I have lost count of the amount of times I have been driving along the road with my head up my arse and the thought of driving head first into a lorry or bus has come in to my head.

It may sound bonkers but that thought has been present many times, I get angry that I've thought like that but at the time the thought feels very much real.

Another scary thought is when I've found myself at the top of a building and the idea of jumping off has been all too common, in reality, thinking straight I know this would never happen because I bloody hate heights and the thought of going even near the edge of a tall building is a big bloody no no.

Another common thought for me is going to sleep and just not waking up, that has always seemed like the best way to stop my anxiety from dragging me down and controlling me, when normal thinking kicks back in I realise that it's the worst bloody thing I can think of as I would be leaving my loved ones behind.

During my numerous trips to see my GP and the other means of help that I have sought, they often ask if I feel or have felt suicidal, I truly believe that I haven't but I do think of ways on which I could end my life, it don't mean I am thinking of doing it, now that's confusing.

People will say you're either suicidal or you're not, that's how anxiety makes you think, irrational twists and turns in your thought process. It doesn't mean I am suicidal, it just means I've had thoughts relating to it.

It's like when they tell you that you're just depressed and need to get out and do more... I get depressed because of my bloody anxiety, if I didn't have this crazy anxiety and think how I do I wouldn't have the bouts of temporary depression.

Which leads me on to my next annoyance, when people tell me I am an angry person, I am not an angry person, I am just so bloody frustrated, but this will make me act and appear an aggressive person but trust me, it's frustration.

This all sounds crazy, doesn't it?

It won't if you suffer like me and just like me you're more than capable of minimising these sort of thoughts, I have now stopped so many of these thoughts before they even start.
It's amazing just how much it makes you realise just how irrational and crazy your thoughts are when you write them down, try it.

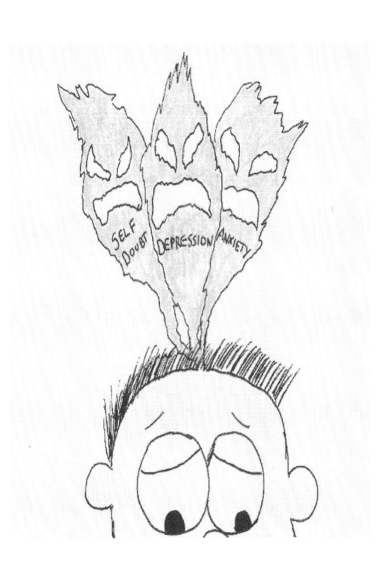

The feeling of being unstable

There is absolutely no question that I can be an unstable person, it's not by choice and virtually everything we feel and worry about when it comes to anxiety links together at some point and this can make us a tad unstable.

Being unstable with my thoughts and behaviour often makes me appear like I have no emotions when it comes to other people's problems or even simple conversations which isn't far from the truth, I am too consumed in my own worry to listen and understand what else is going on around me, this often leads to me becoming angry and yet again frustrated with myself.

Yet again frustration is one of my most common feelings.

CHAPTER SEVEN

I can be such an arsehole

One thing I've definitely been told many times is that I can such an arsehole.

I am often told I am unreasonable and my attitude stinks, the truth be told....it often does

One thing about anxiety is that it will pull us into states where we behave in manners that we don't realise, for many of my anxiety attacks I have probably been unreasonable or in some cases an arsehole to anyone who was around me, that could be in person or even on the likes of social media.

The problem with anxiety is that it effects how we present ourselves to others and frankly we often don't care what we say or think about people at that point in time and in most cases don't even see how we are acting, we are too consumed by what our heading is doing.

Don't get me wrong I am getting better but I often still look back on things I have said or done and think Jesus Bradley that was really arsey or uncalled for.

I get told a lot that I am aggressive or being really negative and I dare say I do come across that way, most of it is frustration around how I am feeling or coping, it is a viscous circle because when people tell you that you're aggressive or negative it just makes you even worse and you become that person they are accusing you of being.

When I look back at my anxiety attacks I will often see that many of them have led to arguments or fights.

I have stormed out of rooms, slammed doors, thrown more things than I care to remember and often screamed or shouted at people, that is once again not being aggressive and crazy, to me it's simply me not coping and losing control.

Some of my outbursts have been over absolutely nothing and it's me that's made a tiny situation a thousand times worse, I really can't empathise enough how fast I used to (and still can) lose control and fly off the handle at people because I wasn't coping or they weren't saying the things I needed to hear, the thing is I didn't even know what I needed to hear so how the hell would they know what to say or do.

I do now find myself apologising on occasion for my attitude and behaviour because I can see it's been over the top and many of the people I have lost control around didn't deserve it.

I often say I don't care what others think and in most cases I don't but there are times where I have been the one at fault and it's important that I hold my hands up and say yup...I was the arsehole and issue any apologies I need too.

Facebook and social media in general can be great for reading and being part of positive things but it also gives us a place to often overreact and come across as someone we really don't mean to be.

I often read some things I have said or posted and shock myself how I have came across, I dare say there will be many more but I am more aware than I once was and instead of hiding from what I've said or I done I will hold up my hands up and say yup....I fucked up.

It's important not to dwell on the times when we fuck up, if you want to apologise then do it and move on, if someone wants to try and make it a bigger issue walk away from the situation and don't let them fuel you, we are far too busy fighting our own issues to let others drag us into bullshit that they feel is important.

Unfortunately, there are people who feed on negativity and will kick others when down, if you feel this is happening then take a step back and remember that you don't have the time for it, let them find another victim.

We have all come across people who love to argue or debate, the smarter one always walks away from that sort of bullshit.

CHAPTER EIGHT

The Everyday Experiences

I could fill this section with dozens and dozens of my anxiety experiences and I am sure you could too but let's focus on my most common as they are the ones that can still catch me by surprise and consume me if I allow them to.

Anxiety does not have set experiences or occasions when it decides to kick in, each and every one of us will have different times that it rears its ugly head but nearly every one of us will most likely act and deal with them the same way.

These experiences are why I have written this book in the first place, I want you to read these with the understanding in your head that I pulled through every single one and I am here telling you about them.

They should be read with the attitude of perhaps relating to them but also realising much of what you suffer personally are false alarms and that you will be fine, if in the future you have a similar experience you can think back to this section and remember I was okay and so will you be.

Caught out in the open and panic sets in

Have you ever walked into a shop or store and all of a sudden you can feel your heart start to race like crazy, your mouth feels dry and you're starting to sweat, there is a sudden feeling of impending doom, you feel like you are struggling to breathe and you need to get out of that place FAST, well that's something that even to this day I often experience, don't get me wrong I have learned to control it far better by using some basic techniques but it still scares the shit out of me until I can get control of the situation.

I have literally had 100s of these bloody attacks, I don't get any warning and thinking back I don't even know why they happened but I do know, like most of my anxiety, they have had a huge impact on even the likes of going shopping.

If I try and think logically why the hell would I be scared of going to perhaps a shop for a new pair of trainers? I shouldn't but by god I have been so many times.

What if I can't get my car parked?

What if the shop is busy and full of people?

What if I see someone I know?

It is amazing just how scared anxiety can and will make you in busy public places and in turn overthink the situation until it escalates out of control.

It wouldn't be the first time that I have driven to the local shopping centre to grab some things and circled the car park and driven back home again because I have just become so overwhelmed and anxious and thought, I'll come back later.

It wouldn't be the first time where I have managed to park the car and walked into the shop and spotted someone I knew and instead of saying hello I have avoided them spotting me and left the shop without getting what I need. This logically makes no sense and it might even be someone I like or know well ,but yup it happens because my head has told me to act in this way and anxiety has taken hold before I could control it and I will often return to my car or avoid the shop until I know they have left.

I still remember an occasion when I was in a store changing room and I heard voices that I recognised outside, anxiety set in and I felt like I was having a meltdown waiting for them to leave so I could come out.

If and when this happens again I try and remember it's yet another attack and that every single one I have experienced in the past was a false alarm and I was fine, I make sure I control my breathing and I try and walk to a location where I can compose myself and take control back.

The important thing is don't fight the attack., your head will always tell you to escape as that's our automatic defence reaction to try and escape the situation or place that you are in, as hard as it will be, try and stay where you are if possible.

Remember to breathe slowly and deeply and the most important thing, as previously mentioned is to **REMIND YOURSELF** that the attack will pass and you will be perfectly fine just like you have been many times before.

Tell yourself that you're not the only one experiencing this and it's a false alarm, in reality there is more than likely other people where you are experiencing these same issues.

Try and focus on something around you or even open up your phone and browse the likes of Facebook or scroll through some pictures of happy memories.

Stay off google, google will tell you what you want to hear and in a state of anxiety your negative thoughts will almost certainly look for negative things on the likes of google, you don't need google, you've been here before and ended up just fine so you will be fine again once this episode passes.

There is no reason why you can't stop the anxiety attack in in its tracks before it takes hold or escalates, you are in control.

Have faith in yourself, it's amazing what just believing in yourself can do to reduce anxiety.

Lack of interest in going places or doing things

I have genuinely lost count on the number of social events or occasions that I have missed or the amount of times I was due to go somewhere but at the last minute changed my mind and ended up staying at home, on many occasions having nothing short of a meltdown and becoming angry that I have let myself and others down, angry that I am missing out.

The problem with Anxiety is that it leaves a lasting effect that can affect your decisions on doing things or going places, on many occasions I have had a night out planned or event to attend and at the last minute my head has taken control and I have decided to not go, that is of course after over thinking for often days or hours on end on the build up to it on reasons why I shouldn't go.

It's almost easier to think of reasons not to go than it is to pull our big boy/girl pants on and go enjoy the event or occasion or at least that's how it seems at the time.

I could tell you about so many times that I have let myself or others down, I have missed everything from family birthdays, work parties to letting my ex-wife and kids down dozens of times and have used every excuse under the sun as to why I haven't gone, excuses seem perfectly acceptable when we are anxious and our minds are made up.

I could probably write a novel purely on excuses I have used over the years or times I have failed to listen to people when they try to help and encourage me to do things with them.

I have lost count on the amount of times I have had someone say to me:

"Just come"

"You will have fun"

"Don't miss this"

"Don't let me down"

"You are being silly"

There is nothing worse than promising someone that you will do something and then letting them down without a genuine reason or in our cases a real reason, anxiety makes you come up all sorts of excuses and lies to avoid going places or doing things.

It hard for me to admit and I have probably never said sorry for the amount of times I have let my ex-wife, kids or friends down by promising to do things with them.

I would promise to take them places and when the day comes around I would either lie that I wasn't feeling well or start an argument or fight so we didn't go, even to this day I can't come up with a valid reason why I wouldn't go other than my head telling me not to.

I have had my kids in tears because I have promised them or their mum screaming at me for letting them down and my head has still taken control I have behaved in a ridiculous manner where nothing they say or do will change how I am thinking, deep down I will hate myself for acting how I am and it often eats me up for days on end but there has been so many times that this has happened and I just can't snap out of it at that point in time.

I think when you have been out in public place and have an attack it leaves a mental scar which can and will make going places or doing things harder and harder, it makes you prepared to let people down to avoid that feeling again but that is the wrong decision to make and only after years of letting people down have I now realised just how unfair and unreasonable I was.

People will tell you to just come or snap out of it…easier said than bloody done, when people try and push you it just leads to even more anxiety and frustration, anxiety has been responsible for me putting many walls up on people that actually do care about me.

The knock on effect with missing events and important occasions is the aftermath of people asking you why you didn't go or wasn't there, on many occasions we will lie and this alone can trigger even more anxiety where I wonder if they know I am lying, are they judging me or do they think I am a failure.

Lack of care for what others has to say

To this day I often ask people a question to be told that they already told me a dozen times or that we have already had this conversation.

I would get angry and demand they tell me again because I can't remember but the truth is that I just wasn't listening or paying attention when they had spoken previously, I am good at that, I am good at "Not Listening" to what others say or ask me, when you're so consumed by your own state of mind you almost flick a switch on what others can be saying or doing around you.

It's not just the going places or doing things that anxiety can ruin, it can put insane pressure on any relationship and frankly I think my family deserves a medal for the absolute lack of interest I have shown when it comes to doing things or even just listening to what they to tell me.
I also have a habit of avoiding conversations that I know will lead to things that I don't want to hear, in my head I have enough issues going on and don't want to add any more, it's easier to avoid conversations and to not engage with people than it is to take part.

There has been an insane amount of times I have been told that I am not interested in what people have to say or asked why I am not giving my view or opinion, the truth is because my head just hasn't let me and I have been just too self-absorbed in myself and my own issues.

I have made huge improvements in engaging and listening, I am not perfect, but it has been great to be part of conversations again and get involved in things, I didn't realise it for many years but having my head think and focus on other things actually helps massively by keeping myself busy with something other than my own thoughts.

If I could say one thing it would be to force yourself to listen to friends, family and loved ones as breaking down and damaging relationships is a hard thing to fix.

Over the years people have often said that I don't reply to messages, phone calls and never speak to them, only looking back do I realise just how bad I was, and it's taken some time to rebuild from how I was.

Having conversations and listening goes hand in hand with allowing ourselves to get out and do more, it's not easy but it is possible, baby steps are better than no steps.

Set small goals to improve on interacting with those around you, even a simple Facebook message to a friend you have not spoken to in a long time can go a long way.

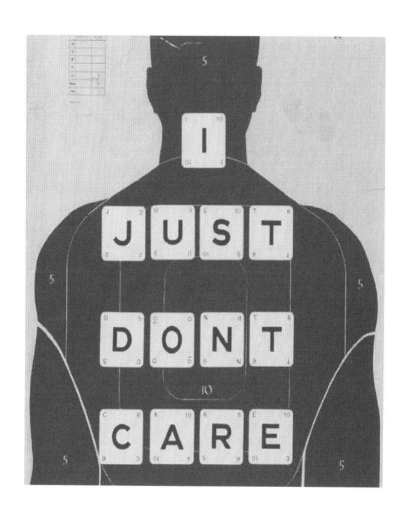

The fear of being ill

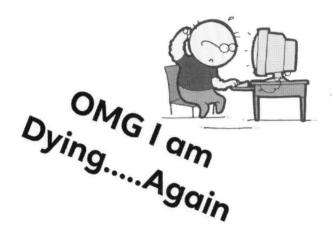

OMG I am Dying.....Again

I genuinely don't think there is an illness that I have not had or at least thought that I had and even now the slightest thing wrong with me will turn in to a huge deal and I'll often be an anxious wreck until it's under control or vanishes.

As far back as I can remember I have always worried about my health, people over the years would laugh and tell me I am such a hypochondriac.

My problem was that I had developed health anxiety and I didn't even realise until things got so bloody crazy and out of control.

There are again 100s of examples I could give but there are a few that really messed me up and at the time I genuinely felt like my life was coming to an end, of course it didn't and again I am here to tell the tale.

I went through a period in my life where I was using sunbeds, I thought I would look better with a tan but it turns out I actually turned orange, but we live and learn.

I was working offshore and to my amazement they had a sunbed we could use, obviously I am not a man to turn down a free sunbed, so I was having a 10-minute session every night for the 2 weeks I was offshore.

Looking back, it was ridiculous, but it was a routine I had gotten myself into.

I remember sitting in my office on the rig when one of the guys passed a comment and said "I am surprised you don't have skin cancer", I laughed it off at the time but it triggered the thoughts about skin cancer and before I knew it was on google reading up on it and any symptoms I might have, one thing google is great at is telling you what you want to hear and if you google for long enough you will find the answers you want to hear or in my case don't want to hear.

It said that moles should be covered up, I have a large mole on my neck and I swear within an hour my whole focus was on the mole on my neck, it was actually feeling pretty sore and looked different to how it used to look, my head start to spin and all of a sudden I started thinking that I had skin cancer.

For the next few days offshore, my head was a mess, I was truly terrified, I couldn't sleep and felt sick all day.
All I could think about was leaving my kids behind.

I could barely focus on my work and a few people asked if I was okay and of course I lied and said I was fine, I couldn't tell them I had cancer as they would laugh or tell me I was being stupid, being told you are stupid when you have anxiety makes things a million times worse.

All I could think about was getting home and getting myself to my doctor, I was sick with worry, my heart was racing virtually all day and I just felt like I had this impending doom hanging over me.

There was a medic offshore, so I decided to go see him to ask if he had anything for the sore head that I was always having, this was 10 years ago, but the experience is still crystal clear in my head.

The medic sat me down and asked a few questions and said let's give you a little check over and he strapped the blood

pressure monitor on to my arm, "that's strange" he said, "let's check it again".
"Bradley, your blood pressure is very high" he said, I felt sick, I asked him why it was so high.

He said "let's check a few other things" and he stuck a heart rate monitor on me, by now I was having one of the biggest attacks I think I have ever had but back then I didn't know this was an anxiety attack, I thought my time was up.

"Bradley your heart rate is through the roof" he said, "I need to call onshore and get some advice", I was panicking, I have never been so close to tears next to another grown man, what is going on, why is this happening was all I could think, this is it for me, my time is up, o-m-g my kids, they need me.

The medic came off the phone and I knew by his face something wasn't right, "Bradley, we need to get you back to Aberdeen" he said.

At that point it was as though my heart had stopped, everything I had worried about was happening, I was going to die.

He told me that they would need to get a chopper from another rig to pick me up and that could take a few hours and to go try and relax and he would call me when he knew when the chopper was due.

I went back to my room and packed my stuff, I couldn't believe what was going on, I was scared, truly scared, the medic had told me not to worry and this was just routine but in my head it wasn't routine and in my head I truly believed that I wouldn't make it back to Aberdeen and to my loved ones.

Once I had packed my stuff I went back to my office and before I knew it I was typing out a letter to my family and my kids, telling them I loved them and telling them the things I was sorry for, I mentioned things like bank account PIN numbers, what to do with my old cars I had...I was writing a will and not a single person to this day, knows how extreme my way of thinking was, I printed it out and put in my bag so if I didn't make it, it would be found.

A few hours passed and the chopper arrived, and I was taken back to Aberdeen where I was met by someone from my company who took me to a medical centre to be checked, I felt overwhelmed that I had made it this far, like it was some sort of achievement that at least I was back in Aberdeen.

When I arrived at the medical centre, I was met by a private doctor who asked some basic questions and took my blood pressure and then my heart rate, he said they are both elevated but not at an amount to cause immediate concern, I felt a slight sense of relief.

He asked if was worrying about anything and as crazy as I knew it would sound I told him about the sunbeds and the mole and my worry about cancer. He took one look at the mole and laughed and said that it was perfectly fine, I told him how it felt sore and he just laughed and said "Bradley, it's fine, it's all in your head", that's a phrase that doctors would tell me a lot over the coming years.

He asked if I was anxious person and if worry a lot and I said "yeah, I worry about absolutely everything", he asked me if I realised that worrying like I do could and would raise my heart rate and blood pressure, I did but when I felt like I did that meant nothing to my train of thought.

He said "Bradley, you are fine, you don't have cancer and I will bet my career that your heart rate and blood pressure is due to you having a serious anxiety attack".

15 mins passed and he took the readings again, "look at that he said, dropping like a stone, you're perfectly fine, less thinking means less worry" he said, "now away you go and relax".

On the way home I took the note out my bag that I wrote for my ex-wife, ripped it up and threw it out of the taxi window, how silly would she think I had been if she found that?

The next day I went to my own GP because as much as the doctor the day before was great I wanted a second opinion, that's one thing about anxiety, we don't always believe what we are told first time round.

I explained what had gone on to my GP and he took both my heart rate and blood pressure, both bang on normal, the sense of relief was overwhelming, I hated that I had felt how I did for the last 24 hours but at the same time I was able to accept it was all in my head.

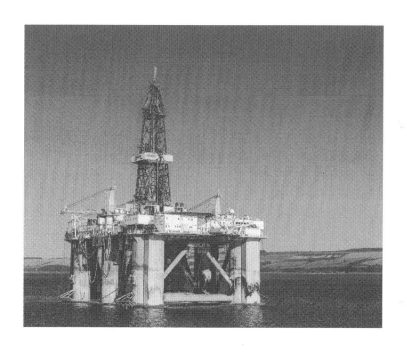

A typical North Sea Oil Rig

I am having a heart attack

Let's be clear, I have never had a heart attack but on many occasions I sure as hell thought I was and have ended up at Accident and Emergency telling them I was.

For years I have experienced chest pains and my head has taken control and I have been convinced I am having or about to have a heart attack.

Looking back, it's ridiculous that I was able to drive myself to accident and Emergency, if I had truly been having a heart attack there was no way I would have been able get in a car and drive, but all normal thinking goes out of the window when we have these attacks.

There has been loads of occasions where this has happened but looking back, one definitely sticks out and is the one I look back to remind me that most of what I think is just in my head.

For a quite few weeks I had been experiencing pains in the left side of my chest that would come and go but the feelings of worry would not shift, I just kept thinking something wasn't right and the pains seemed to be getting worse, I had no idea what was causing them and as the weeks went on the worry was turning into panic, like most times I was on google and looking for clues and of course everything was pointing to a heart problem or at least it was in my head.

Pains in the chest were key symptoms of people who have had heart attacks and my head was now focused badly on my heart, looking back I ignored all the other symptoms I was experiencing.

One thing anxiety does is make us fixate on things and believe them and that day I truly believed I was having a heart attack.

I had been to the gym and had come home, my ex-wife and kids were out so I was alone in the house, the pains in my chest seemed for stronger than normal and my heart was starting to race, I was now becoming short of breath, the more I focused on my chest and heart racing the more frantic I became and before I knew it was on my way to accident and emergency.

When I arrived I told the girl on the desk that I was having chest pains and before I knew it was whisked away by a nurse who took me into a room and asked me all sorts of questions, she took my heart rate and blood pressure, "they are both really high" she said, now I know I have had issues with these before thanks to previous anxiety attacks but at the time I didn't tell her and not because I had forgotten but because I didn't want to tell her about them and not be taken seriously.

I was taken through to a ward and told a doctor would be with me shortly, they strapped a machine to my chest which I have now know is called an ECG machine.

The nurse said don't worry we are keeping an eye on you, I was hooked up to various machines and she left.

I remember laying there thinking 'why aren't they doing something?', 'why has she just left me here when I could die at any moment', sounds crazy but that's how my mind was thinking.

There was a huge sense of relief that I was in the right place and that they would come running if one of the machines started making noises, I remember staring at the machines looking for changes on what they were saying and listening to every noise they made but in reality I had no idea what any of it meant

After what felt like a decade (but it was probably about 40 minutes) a doctor arrived and sat next to me and said, "so what's going on then?".

I told him that I had been having chest pains and that my heart rate and blood pressure were high, he looked across at the machine that connected to me and said "well, your heart rate is fine now, let me take your blood pressure again".
He took my blood pressure and said "it's normal" both had dropped back to normal levels since I had first seen the nurse.

He took a look at the results from the ECG tracing that the nurse had done and said they look good.

He said "let's do a quick once over" so he started by feeling my stomach and side and moved up to my chest, as he pressed down on my left side of my chest there was a shooting pain and I almost leapt off the bed.

"Well that's a good sign" he said…good sign… it was bloody sore and proved I was having chest pains.

He focused on the left-hand side of my chest and every so often I would get a pain when he pushed down on it.

"I know what the issue is, Bradley", my heart almost stopped with worry.

"Your ECG is fine and so are your heart rate and blood pressure, in fact everything looks great, but you have pulled a muscle in your chest and that's why you are having pains", I didn't know whether to should laugh or cry.

The treatment…2 ibuprofen and to lay off the gym for a few days, another case of Anxiety 1 – Bradley 0

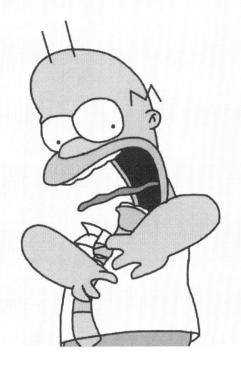

I went through what felt like a decade where I had constant sore throats and no matter what I tried they just kept coming back.

I was eating packs of sore throat sweets daily, but it turns out the sugar in the them actually dries your throat out even more.

Anyone who has experienced a sore throat that won't go away can tell you just how much it can get you down, this drove me into a horrible place as people would tell me "it's just a sore throat", trust me, nothing is ever "just a sore throat" when you are an anxious person.

The feeling of my throat feeling tight and sore to swallow is something for a long time I could not shift nor could I understand why it kept coming back.

The problem is when you have been visiting your doctor for so many other reasons something like a sore throat makes you almost embarrassed to visit them for.

Eventually I did visit my local GP who inspected my throat which had a horrible yellow gunk inside it and over my tongue; I was told it looked like a throat infection and given antibiotics for two weeks but I suspect he knew it was anxiety but knew I would doubt him so medication would send me away in a better frame of mind, he was right.

I started taking the medication but in my head I was convinced it was pointless and the doctor had got it wrong, nearly every time I go to the doctor I think they have got it wrong and something serious is going to happen, funnily enough it never does.

Two weeks passed and it did feel and look much better and my anxiety and worry had almost gone completely, I was cured…

The problem was a month or so later it was back, back to where I started, back to the doctor I went and this time around I was given a throat spray to try and although it did make it ease off and more comfortable it didn't make it go away, by now I was overthinking my throat issues to the maximum and it was really getting me down.

In my head I had throat cancer and back on google this was confirming my worries, back to my GP I went and this time I told him how I was thinking and although he did brush off what I was telling him he did say he would take a swab of my throat and send it off for checking.
Sounds great that he was having the swab tested but when you're kept waiting for results your head makes the already bad situation so much worse.

A week of absolute hell passed, and the results came back, no infection, no issues and yup…no cancer.

I was called back in to see my GP and he started speaking about me being an anxious person who worries a lot, this was becoming a theme, every time I was going to the doctor he was now blaming or mentioning anxiety.

He went on to explain that a sore throat is one of the most common side effects of anxiety and elevated stress levels are the cause.

I liked what I heard but of course I doubted him because that's what we do.

Since then I often get sore throats, in fact if I think and worry about a sore throat long enough, I will get one but at least now I am normally able to get it under control before it gets worse.

My throat is always at its worst when I have a heightened state of stress or I am feeling anxious but at least now I can almost ignore the throat part and fixate on what else the anxiety is doing to me, how stupid does that sound?

There have been so many other things have happened over the years that at the time felt like there was no way out and my time was coming to an end, but yet I am still here.

CHAPTER NINE

I forget what sleep is like

I am so tired anxiety and poor sleep go hand in hand and I genuinely can't remember the last time I had a solid night sleep.

There is no doubt that anxiety can and will fuel insomnia for many of us.

If I am not fighting trying to get to sleep in the first place I am tossing and turning the entire night.

Most people go to bed to sleep, I go to bed to turn my head on and think about absolutely everything and anything, this is not by choice.

It's been a common occurrence to be sitting on the edge of my bed virtually in tears with the frustration.

I have taken part in sleep studies, I have tried virtually every sleeping medication known to man and although there have been periods where medication has worked I sooner or later get used to what I am taking, and the broken sleep and dread of bed time soon returns.

I have lost count of the amount of times I have lashed out at my ex-wife in the middle of the night because she has shouted at me or complained because I was keeping her up. It's wasn't ex-my wife's fault and she was entitled to her sleep but in the middle of the night when I was drained, frustrated and on the verge of self-destruction whatever she said was never accepted and it was all too easy to blame her or lash out.

For months on end I would sleep in the spare room to avoid waking up my kids, I would enter the room and close the door and it's then just me and my thoughts to battle it through the night.

At my worst, the thoughts that would enter my head were often scary and like the work of anxiety they were beyond irrational.

When the lack of sleep goes on for months and in my case years on end, bed time becomes a scary thought and I for many years dreaded it, worrying about not being able to sleep makes bed time a stressful and fearsome time.

In fact, 90% of this book has been written when I should be sleeping and simply didn't know what to do, this was my way of stopping me lying in bed becoming agitated and frustrated.

Like I have mentioned previously lack of sleep and anxiety go hand in hand and lack of sleep can massively affect your mood the next day or for the days to come.

Entering each day exhausted and mentally drained is one of the worst feelings and I have often felt like I was ready to have some sort of breakdown, I felt like I was going crazy as it sucks everything from you.

I have left quite a few jobs over the years due to my anxiety, but sleep deprivation definitely played a part on me either not turning up or simply giving up on trying to function at my place of work.

My sleep is slightly better thanks to my GP helping with changing out my medication when they no longer become effective but it's far from perfect, I still have many nights where sleep just doesn't happen, and I enter the next day drained and exhausted.

The biggest help to me was forcing myself to stop worrying about the next day and not being able to function for the likes of work, forcing myself to turn off all gadgets and set myself a strict rule for lights out and head down has definitely helped, it is far from perfect but it's getting better.

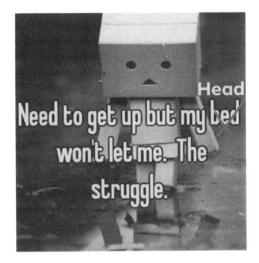

CHAPTER TEN

Accepting who I am

I have accepted that in my head I have multiple health issues but virtually all of them come from my anxiety, there is no doubt in my mind and I have now accepted that in the past this has led to bouts of depression, this book, writing and reading it has played a huge part in me accepting my issues.

Daily I still fight the battle of anxiety and in turn my mental health can still be unstable, until about a year ago when I started writing this book you would never hear me say or admit that.

It took a bloody long time to realise that the cure sits within myself and how I deal with each and every occurrence of my anxiety, there are of course ways to help but ultimately it comes down to me…it comes down to us and it can be done.

When I look back at the number of things I did to try and rid myself of my anxiety it blows my mind, I did everything these books told me to do, I had numerous sessions with experts and my GP was borderline on speed dial, so why am I not "fixed"?

I kept hearing the same message that every day is a new day and to just push past it and it will get better but it wasn't getting better, it was getting worse, my head was exploding.

Every bloody day all I could think about was:

Why am I like this?
Why do I feel like I do?
Why am I always so anxious and drained for
no reason at all?
Why is this happening to me?

I still often sit and think to where this all began and at what point anxiety entered my life.

When I was growing up, I had never heard of anxiety so if I did have issues then it wasn't diagnosed or addressed, in fact I didn't really know or understand what anxiety was until around 10 years ago when things led to me visiting my GP for help on the things I was feeling and issues I was having.

Doctors can be great, and I think they do an amazing job based on the time they have and just like every job they are limited based on their experience.
I have lost count of how many GP's I have seen and the crazy amount of times I have made appointments when feeling at my worst and felt I had nowhere else to turn.

When the appointments came around I didn't even turn up as on the day I simply self-destructed, anxiety took over and I convinced myself not to go...Stupid move, Bradley

Google and Self Diagnosing

Instead I would sit at home and sit on the likes of google, self-diagnosing and looking for answers, the problem with google is that it has an answer for absolutely everything and that is both good and bad.

When you have an anxious frame of mind and are searching for answers the likes of google will throw up both the good and bad and without fail, we focus in on the bad…it's what we do.

If you remember one thing from this section, remember Google is a machine, it will tell you whatever you want it to and you won't believe it.
If you do want use google I found that finding a select few sites that have worked for you previously were the ones to bookmark and only visit them, don't go searching for more and more answers, it won't help.

There are some great forums that I've joined and often read when I want to give myself a reminder that I am not alone, I often read other people's problems and issues and it can instantly make me feel 100 times better and get me thinking straight again, on many occasions we will chat away in groups…Finally people wo understand.

It took many years but accepting that I had anxiety was hard when I didn't understand what it actually was but after the doctors' appointments, the relating to what other people online were experiencing I finally accepted what I have but that was only the beginning.

Google

| is Evil | ✕ | 🔍 |

Search On: Using tech for cleaner water

CHAPTER ELEVEN

Living with a secret

For a man that's just written a book about anxiety, until very recently it was a secret that I hid from many until I realised just how many of us suffer from it, it is said that in our lifetime 1 in 4 of us will suffer anxiety at some point, many of us long term.

Social media and the likes make removing stigmas so much easier these days and it is also powerful for surrounding yourself with people who perhaps suffer with the same things you do and can help you to gain a greater understanding of your feelings.

Let's face it, everyone has secrets but many of us live with the fact we have Anxiety and choose to keep it a secret, bad choice.

Reasons why we think we should keep it as a secret.

- What If my employer finds out
- I feel so embarrassed
- People will think I am weak
- He/she is lying
- They are such an attention seeker
- I won't get invited places by friends
- Everyone thinks I am a burden

It's easier to make excuses as to why you should keep it a secret than it is to just be open and honest when the time arises.

It is already a huge effort battling anxiety and keeping it at bay, fighting it, suppressing it and keeping it a secret will only feed it and make it grow.

So many of us are already under huge pressure perhaps at work or at home with loved ones or perhaps the growing up of our children, perhaps there are other worries at home, you may not realise it, but anxiety is adding to them.

We spend so much time trying to impress people at work, appearing happy and healthy on the likes of social media or pushing for that perfect relationship or even just trying to fit in.

It is amazing just how many other people may be experiencing what you are and battling their own struggles and demons.

Anxiety picks absolutely anyone, the guy in the shop, your boss at work, even the doctor who you often visit.

The best and most rewarding thing I ever did was get mine out there in the open and in turn write this book to remind not only myself but also you that we are not alone and most of what we feel is the work of our head playing cruel tricks on us.

It is okay to not be okay and by god you'll be amazed at how much relief you get my getting that weight off your shoulders.

If people ask me how I am and it feels appropriate I'll be often be open and honest, it might just be that I've had a shit few months and that my anxiety has been pretty wild but I'm pushing to keep beating it, sometimes that simple conversation opens up a bigger conversation and often leads to a sense of getting it off your chest.

Don't suffer in silence and remember people are understanding and compassionate but you need to give them that chance.

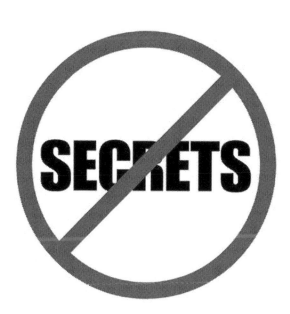

CHAPTER TWELVE

Seeking help

There is no question that we shouldn't suffer alone and many of us will find support using difference means but seeking help is key and in turn use that to learn about your illness.

I found on many occasions that I would leave my GP more anxious and frustrated than I was when I went in but looking back that was because I either had a wall up and wasn't being honest with him or I was simply expecting too much and hoping to leave with some miracle cure, I have lied to my GP in hope of getting medication because at the time that's what my head told me I needed to be "fixed"

The hardest but most important part about visiting any doctor is to try and be open and honest but also get across what you want to say or speak about, this can be tough as we always have a million things in our heads to say or ask but on the day very few come out.

If and when I visit my GP, I now write down what I want to say, this could be one or two points, or it could be a list of worries that have been playing havoc with me.

I often laugh about it but it's like a shopping list of things that I want to say or ask and the difference it has made to my GP appointments has been transformational.

I can now get so much more out of my GP visits but he can also gain so much more of an understanding of how I am thinking and he is able to prioritise any help I might need or even just engage in a conversation that helps because let's face it, a good solid, understanding conversation from someone such as GP makes a huge difference for us.

CBT

Most GP's will try and suggest trying an individual self-help course to see if it can help you learn to cope with your anxiety.

I've tried CBT courses but I just couldn't make them work for me, but they are definitely worth trying and do allow you to get down on paper things that are going on your head and help you to start to understand yourself a bit more, enter anything such as CBT courses with an open mind.

Medication

One thing that doctors are quick to hand out is medication, at first, I would take absolutely anything if it would help and more so in my later years of my Anxiety where every day was a train wreck.

Medication does have its place and has worked for millions of people so also enter that with an open mind, I still take medication daily which has definitely helped once I eventually found what worked for me but it did take years of trial and error before I found something that has helped but that didn't come without its price and that price was Diazepam which left me at one point with an addiction and in serious trouble.

Diazepam

This is where things went horribly wrong for me when it comes to medications.

Diazepam although prescribed in fairly low doses is habit forming, of course I didn't know that at the time and these little blue pills when taken, would make me feel calm and generally in a far nicer place, the problem was I was taking them far more than advised, if I felt the slightest bit of anxiety kicking in I would take one and they would take the edge off how I was feeling.

Within no time one pill did nothing and I was doubling the dose, without realising I was becoming addicted, it got to the point where I had run out and my GP made it clear that he could not issue me anymore, this sent my anxiety soaring like never before, I didn't know what to do.

I found a page online that was offering them on the black market and although in my head I knew this was a ridiculous idea, before I knew it I had purchased a large quantity of tablets which were 5 times the dosage my GP had given me.
My head was telling me I could break the tablets up and keep the dose low just like my GP had given but in reality, this didn't happen.

Over the period of around 2 years I used Diazepam to numb the bouts of Anxiety and thoughts in my head, when

I look back now, I realise I was doing no such thing, I was actually fuelling my anxiety with an addiction and actually making myself and sanity worse than ever.
As soon as I woke each day, I would take a Diazepam, looking back I wasn't even giving myself a chance to start the day positive.

Some days I would take up to 10 tablets and at my lowest I would walk around in a daze not enjoying anything or anyone I was with.
I was a particularly bad person to be around and at this stage, I was now a paranoid wreck.
I seldom left the house until I was almost forced to do so, the strain on my marriage was at breaking point and I had to do something before I lost my entire world or worse…my life

I was terrified to speak to my GP but as the weeks went past I decided that I needed to take action and booked an appointment to see him.

The day of the appointment arrived, and I was nothing short of frantic, what was I going to say to him?
I have let him down, I have let myself down, and what will he say?

Where do I even start when I walk into his room and what do I say?

In my head my issues are all over the place, I am abusing drugs and my mental state terrifies me, maybe I just shouldn't go and just keep taking the drugs that I am now buying from local drugs dealers or absolutely anywhere I could get my hands on them.

I take some Diazepam and the calmness kicks in which was enough to let me travel to the appointment, as I enter the waiting room I can feel my face start to heat up and my heart is racing faster and faster, the palms of my hands have become all clammy and I start to panic, I sit down and try to control my breathing.

I start to play about on my phone, I read the posters on the wall and I pick up some magazines about gardening, I hate bloody gardening but I flick through the pages, my name is shouted and I swear to god my heart nearly stopped.
We enter his room and he asks me to take a seat, I felt physically sick.

By now I am terrified and it was obvious as he could see it, he asks me to calm down and proposes have a chat about why I am back to see him as he thought everything was better as I'd not been to see him in many months.

At first it was like someone had frozen my head and my thoughts, I couldn't get out the dozens of things in my head that I had been thinking on the way to my appointment that I wanted to, but more importantly needed to tell him.

Eventually I blurted it out, I've been taking diazepam that I bought off the internet and I can't cope anymore.
I told him how I hated my life and don't see any purpose anymore and that my thoughts terrified me.

I don't want to be here, I don't want to feel the way I do, I had tears in my eyes, and I felt sick, my heart was pounding, and I could feel myself struggling to breathe. The last time I cried was about 20 years earlier when my gran died, I am deep person, crying isn't something I do, I was embarrassed, I just wanted to run out of the room but he was great and just calmly said "don't worry you are in the right place, take your time".

He went on to tell me that I was not alone in what I had done and that he could help, straight away he told me he didn't suffer from anxiety so he wouldn't bullshit me that he did but what he did say is that he could help me understand myself and start to look at how we could make things better, he had never spoken like that before, I instantly felt a weight being lifted.

He then went on to tell me certain scenarios that hit me like a brick, everything he said I had at some point went through.

He said we wouldn't fix how I was overnight and that it was a slow process but we could put things in place to try and manage what I experienced, I liked this guy, I like he was honest and not bullshitting me.

He made it clear the diazepam had to stop, we put a plan in place on how to slowly come off what I was taking and introduce something less habit forming.

For the next 15 mins we spoke about many things, most of which wasn't even about my anxiety, it was about happy things, happy moments in my life, this guy was smart, I felt like someone was listening, someone was understanding, he then said "think about what we just spoke about, you have many great things in your life and we can push to make many more".

We agreed I would go back in a month to see how coming off the diazepam had gone and if I had managed we would put a plan in place for me, I told him I hate reading and listening to things as they didn't work and often made me feel worse, he agreed that my plan would be something I owned and was responsible for and he will help me where he could.

A month went past and every single time I had a feeling that I needed diazepam I remembered how my GP was and the time he gave me to listen and offer to help, it worked and 4 weeks later I was back and no diazepam had been taken in a number of days.

He told me he wanted to try me on another drug called Trazadone which can be taken long term with little to no side effects, he then told me that at any point if I need someone to speak to then he was just around the corner, he gave me some material that he had hand written just for me, he knew I hated reading things that were over complicated or written by someone who I couldn't relate to, the fact he took the time out to do that for me was very overwhelming.

I had a plan, I left his office with the sense I could do this for the first time in as long as I could remember.

Since that day I have been back and forth to my GP and some private GP appointments when I have lost control and felt like I had nowhere to turn but nothing like the number of visits I used to have.

I stayed on the drug Escitalopram for around 2 years and stopped taking it when I felt like I had gained some control and learned much of what I have spoken about in this book.

Learning the triggers and learning ways to control my issues is what has helped me on the way to recovery, I still have my issues and have the odd relapse but I have learned to accept that, I no longer dwell on them and my goal is to look in front of me, never behind.

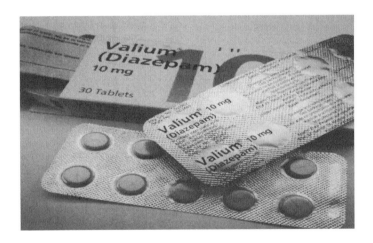

CHAPTER THIRTEEN

Coping Mechanisms

There are many theories on how to stop the thoughts brought on by anxiety, so I have listed a few that I have used and have definitely helped over the years.

The thing to remember is that as long as you have anxiety you're going to be more open to thoughts that can trigger many other emotions.

Anxiety changes the chemistry in the brain and will make it easier for the mind to focus on the negative or scary thoughts that can consume you.

You are more likely to have a scary thought when you have anxiety and you are also more likely to focus on the thought and then have the thought cause more even more anxiety.

You need to control your anxiety and not let it control you, you are going to need to find ways to avoid worrying about the thoughts as much.

Keeping yourself busy or surrounding yourself with people you enjoy being around is the first choice for me, I used to avoid doing things and being around people but that is not the answer, I now go out of my way to force myself to do things and by god, what a difference it's made.

Some ways to help cope when everything else seems to fail:

Write the Thought Down

The mind is more likely to stop focusing on something scary when it has it written down in a permanent place. When these thoughts are distressing you, write the thought down in a log, I use the notepad on my phone but then again, I use it for many notes and virtually this entire book was written on my iPhone notes section.

The next time you have an attack you can look back and remind yourself you have been here before and was perfectly fine, a little bite can give big reassurance.

Accept the Thoughts

We have already covered this, but you are also going to need to accept that these thoughts occur and happen. While they may distress you, the more you try to fight them the worse they can become.

It's in your best interests to be okay with the fact that you have these thoughts and that alone is part of the cure, accept you know you have anxiety and these thoughts are going to happen.

Anything that distracts you from negative thoughts can be valuable, especially if it's positive.

Consider funny shows on television or try calling a friend, obviously a happy one and not one that is prone to sucking the life out of you, we all have one of those.

CHAPTER FOURTEEN

Thinking about Anxiety don't have to be scary

I used to be terrified of writing or even thinking about my Anxiety for the fear of making myself worse and the truth be told, I used to scare myself into having even more attacks when I did.

It took me a long time to learn to be able to think about my anxiety without having a meltdown or losing even more control.

Writing this book was always going to be a huge challenge as it was going to make me think and face many of the issues I have faced.

I am sat writing this very chapter on a plane on the way back from an amazing family holiday in Florida, I hate flying, everything about it makes me anxious and I will do absolutely anything to make the flight pass quicker, this flight I am using this book as my pass quicker plan.

There is no doubt that Anxiety is fuelled and made worse by over thinking and in nearly all cases it has been the reason I've lost control on many occasions when I've thought about previous episodes.

When I now start to think of my past attacks, I also bust my ass to think of the positives and how eventually I was okay.

In the build up to this family holiday in Florida I worked myself into a frenzy about the plane journey and trip itself, I even took a trip to my GP as I just couldn't get into my head that I would be okay flying and also had a terrible fear that something would happen to me when I was away, this wasn't just about flying, I was thinking about every irrational thing I could wrong on the build up to going away.

My head was telling me the plane was going to crash, it was telling me that I was going to get a blood clot on the plane and have a huge heart attack, when I got to Florida I was going to take ill and my kids would have to watch this happen, it terrifies me that they would witness this happen and I just couldn't shift it from my head and thoughts.

My GP did his usual speech but in my head all I wanted was some drugs that I could take to calm my thoughts if they did escalate out of control before I even got on the plane.

My GP is great and he agreed to give me 4 diazepam, 2 before the flight and 2 for after, not very much but it was enough to calm me ever so slightly knowing I had that safety net, I did ask why just 4 and he said "Bradley, we have been here before, you don't need them, go have a great holiday and remember that you can control your thoughts better than you previously could".

Funnily enough I made it to Florida and the plane didn't crash but I was far from out of the woods.

On the first day I read a post on Facebook about someone who has spotted a snake in their hotel, I hate snakes and this set off a frenzy of worrying thoughts and anxiety about encountering a snake and being bitten by it.
Little do my kids know but every single day I was looking for snakes, at bed time I would search the apartment from top to bottom, all without them, I needed to make sure no snakes had sneaked in, needless to say I never found one and thinking about it, if I had found one I would have been out of that room before they even knew what was going on.

Dad is a pussy

On holiday I must have been mocked and called a pussy by my oldest son at least a hundred times, it was all in fun but one thing I hate is heights and things I don't have control of...Roller coasters are up there on my 'stay the hell away from list.'

I managed to avoid many of the roller coasters and had to sit and watch my 11,12 and 19 year old kids go on them while Dad the pussy sat them out....but I didn't avoid them all and there was a few I was dragged on to almost kicking and screaming, I am no expert but Jesus I looked these things up and down and looked at every component my eyes would allow....looking for something wrong but surprisingly I found nothing and although my heart raced like crazy and I was convinced I was about to become another statistic, here I am telling you all about it....I survived it, albeit a pussy

When not at the theme parks my friend Anxiety like back home was always lurking and I did have various attacks over the two weeks which would range from the fear of crashing the hire car to someone stealing our entire holiday spending money from the room safe and us being left with nothing and a ruined holiday, all vey real feelings at the time.

Learning from my past mistakes

It's only after many years of ruining special occasions and family trips that I now know that having these attacks on holiday are the last thing my family want or need to hear.

It is brutally hard to not tell those around you what you're thinking when it's your loved ones but there is a time and a place and a family trip away isn't one of them, when I did have these attacks I would try and minimise them by whatever means I could and the best tactic for me was to simply focus on things that made me smile that day, I would look at pictures we had taken or I would look at ideas for what we could do the following day or even just sit and remind myself about my thousands of attacks I have had and how I was always fine at the end of each, sitting here on the plane I am rather proud of myself that I didn't just beat the most of the attacks from escalating whilst away but I stopped myself ruining my family's trip and memories.

If I could give one piece of advice, and I know it's by no means easy, it would be to remember those around us are entitled to be okay and have fun even when we are struggling, remember if they are okay and happy then so can we be, feed on their joy and mood, it's amazing how much it can help a situation be so much easier or stop it totally.

If we go back to what this chapter is about, I have managed to cover some of what I worried about and had issues with while on holiday and here I am telling you, a huge achievement alone for me.

The plane didn't crash, there was no roller coaster issues and absolutely everything I thought at the time was one big false alarm, writing them down did give me some flash backs but I haven't avoided thinking about them, don't be scared to think about past anxiety attacks, if you are thinking about your past issues it means you beat them and you are here reminding yourself that.

I will say this many times throughout this book but admitting to ourselves what we suffer is the first step to controlling much of what we suffer and think.

It is not easy, but it can be done even in tiny steps.

I will have more attacks and I will share them with you, there is absolutely no doubt about that, but I will also share how I beat them.

CHAPTER FIFTEEN

Never give up

I have shared just some of my anxiety attacks over the years and my challenging times that I have endured in my life.

Out of all that events I have now been able to grasp an understanding of my anxiety and learn from it, I've learnt to now not let it consume me and I truly believe you can too.

No matter what, you need to learn to control your anxiety and more importantly believe you can

I have become aware that my irrational thoughts were mostly the cause of my anxiety and not necessarily the situations at hand, I have been able to disregard these patterns of thinking that seemed to be the catalyst for all these episodes.

I refuse to dwell on the past event and simply learn from it, nothing good comes from negative thinking, negative or fearful thoughts, all these do is generate stress and anxiety

Hopefully like me, you may now recognise these patterns of thinking and know they can be and most likely are, the triggers for your anxiety, knowing what's going on within your head is incredibly powerful.

Whenever I feel an episode of anxiety starting to come on, I simply know that my thinking is nonsense at this point I simply try and stay in control and remind myself that we have been here before, remind myself it is a false alarm.

Today I still have plenty worry and often my fear and anxiety creeps back, but I feel like I truly understand it now and I can see what caused me so many issues over the years.

The patterns of thinking and believing the irrational thoughts that come in to my head are mostly ignored now.

I have beaten this, I tell myself this daily and it has worked wonders for me.

If during an attack you start to react with fear or have that feeling of needing to escape remind yourself that your symptoms are just a false alarm that and they can and will vanish as quickly as they started.

Your plan is to not just beat anxiety but to also control it, when you learn to do that, you'll regain control back of your head, health and in turn get your life back to where you want it.

The more people that talk about their issues and the sooner we remove the stigma, the more people will seek help.

The next time you have an attack, remember 3 key points:

Recognise:

The next time you notice increased anxiety or panic symptoms, simply pause and take a breath.
Take this moment to recognise that you are experiencing anxiety.
Acknowledging your symptoms at the start of a panic attack can give you a sense of power over your fears and kick it in the ass before it takes hold, I have now stopped many attacks before they started and so can you.

Accept:

Rather than trying to run away from or resist your symptoms, learn to recognise the attack.

Acceptance doesn't mean that you're giving in to panic, but it will provide you with the thoughts you need to get through the attack and stop it.

Remind:

Don't allow yourself to become wrapped up in fear, remind yourself that these are symptoms of a panic attack that are not new to you and that you have nothing to be afraid of as you've beaten many before.

Closing Words

People often ask me if I am cured of anxiety now that I have been able to speak about it and write this book. I am certainly not cured but I have managed to stop many attacks that in the past would have brought me to my knees.

I have so much to live for and so do you.
Giving up is not an option and although our head often tells us that we can't go on, I have learned and often remind myself that we can.

I would definitely say this book has helped me find myself and made me understand who I am as person. I seldom run to my doctor like I did for many years and when I feel like I can't perform or do things I push myself to remember the times when everything has been fine, and I made it through that day. In fact, I remind myself of the happy times and good feelings when I don't have anxiety, being positive is what I now believe has kept many anxiety attacks from even starting to happen in the first place.

I used to be terrified of speaking about my anxiety or reading about other people's issues. I have now reversed that way of thinking to remind myself that speaking up and hearing how other people are means that I am not alone and that many of us have issues, there is no shame in feeling how we often do.

I know it's tough and you may have felt that you can't go on and see no way out, there is a way out and you can and will get better. I often thought that anxiety was so powerful that it controlled me and many times it did, but I now know I can control it.

I am in charge and although it's by no means easy, we can definitely take more control of the situations we find ourselves in.

I no longer look for a quick fix or the cure that I wanted for many years. I understand what I have and instead of being scared of it I now continually remind myself how far I have come, and I would like you to learn and feel the same. I know you can do it too.

I have given myself goals to achieve in my career and promised to be a stronger person for my family and friends, I really believe I can do that.

I really hope this book has helped you being able to walk my journey with me.

We all have it in us to feel better and take control of our issues.

Don't set yourself a time to feel better and lessen your anxiety, take it as it comes, and you can always pop back to this book for that reminder that you will be okay and you can beat this.

All the best.

Bradley

Good luck, you can beat this and remember……

ITS OK TO NOT BE OK

A selection of pictures over the years of some happy times

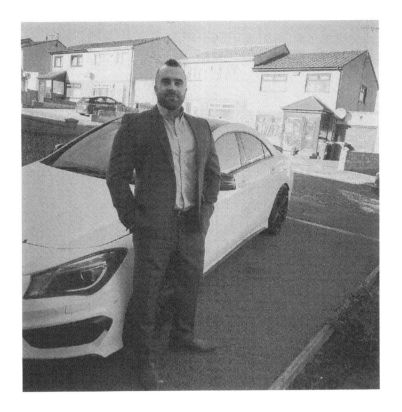

Bradley Feb 2019

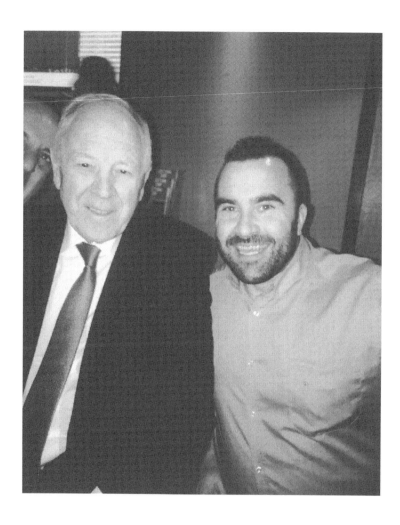

Bradley and Craig Brown former Scotland FC
Manager

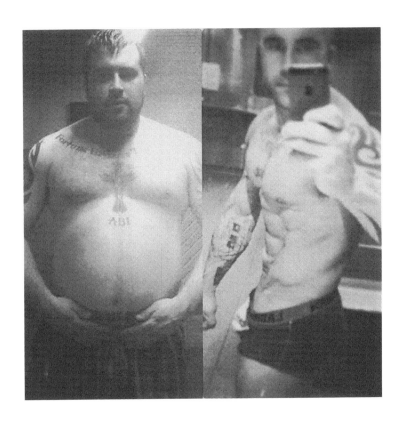

My weight loss Journey 2009 vs 2015

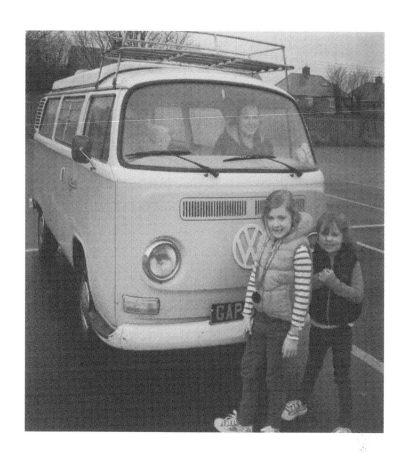

Family trip in 2011 a classic VW camper

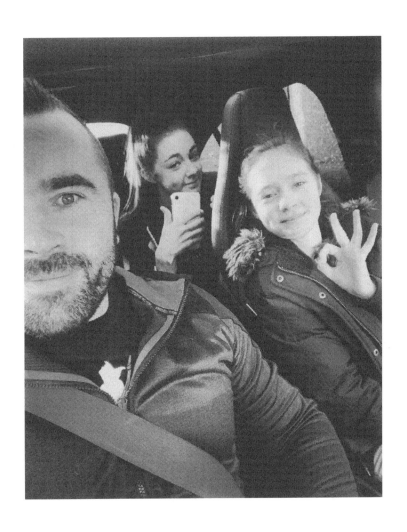

Bradley and his children Dec 2018

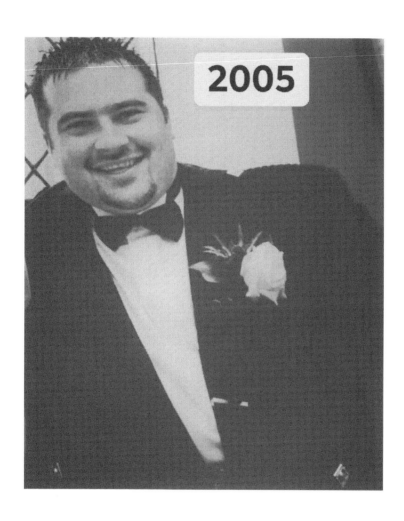

Bradley in 2005

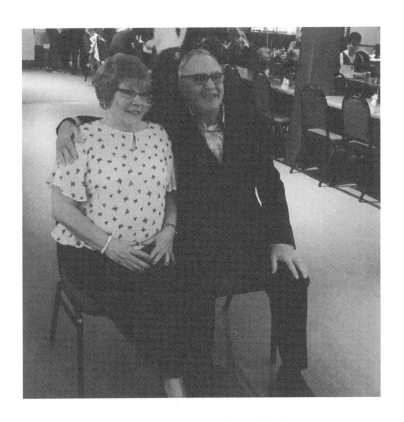

Bradleys Mums 70th Birthday 2018

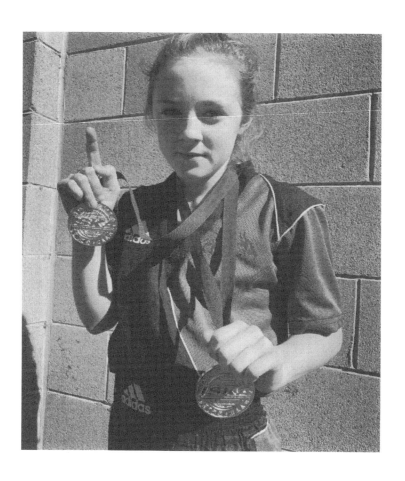

My daughter, 12 years old at the time of writing and both Scottish and British Kickboxing champion in 2017

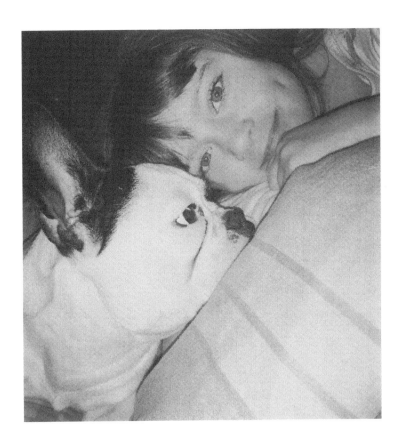

Bradleys youngest daughter with their French Bulldog Frank.

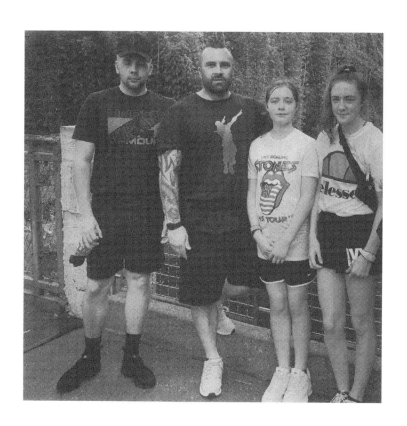

Bradley and his children, Florida 2018

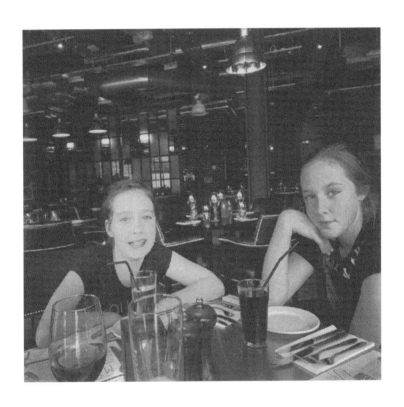

Bradleys daughters Edinburgh 2017

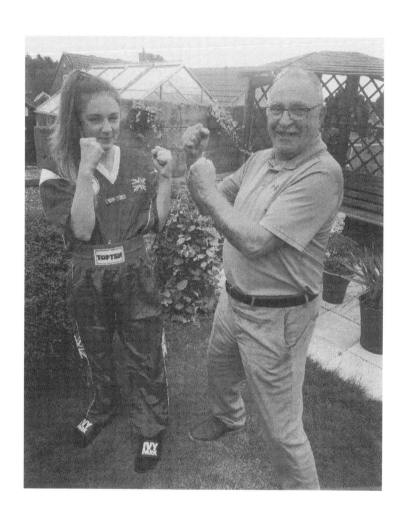

Bradleys daughter and his father 2018

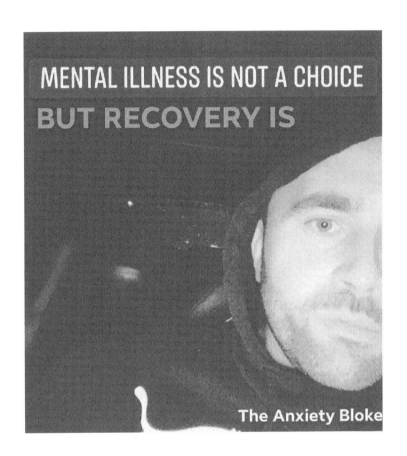

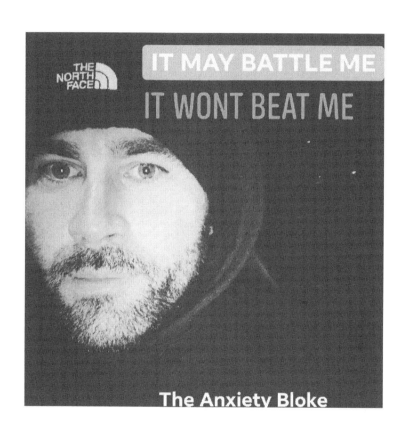

BE A WARRIOR
NOT A WORRIER

The Anxiety Bloke

TIME WILL PASS
THESE FEELINGS WILL PASS
AND EVENTUALLY...
I will be myself again

TheAnxietyBloke

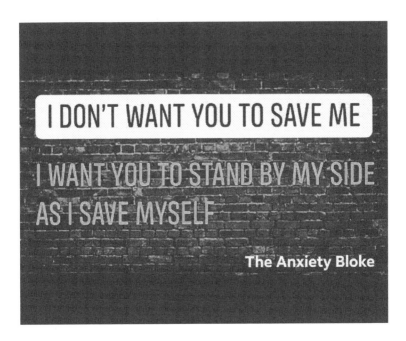

I DON'T WANT YOU TO SAVE ME

I WANT YOU TO STAND BY MY SIDE
AS I SAVE MYSELF

The Anxiety Bloke

About the Author:

Bradley currently resides in Aberdeen, Scotland and has 3 children.

Career driven and has worked from everything from a bin man to a company director.

Bradley when not with his family enjoys the gym and modifying cars or anything with an engine.

A typical family man who has overcome many battles when it comes to Anxiety but like many of us still faces them on occasion.

A strong believer in what doesn't beat us will make us stronger and is passionate about helping others.

Facebook: www.facebook.com/theanxietybloke
Instagram: @theanxietybloke
Email: bradley@theanxietybloke.com

Anxiety has taken control of my life...**I admit that.**
Anxiety has made me a liar... **I admit that but I am getting better.**
Anxiety has made me a crap person to be around... **I admit that.**
Anxiety has made me unapproachable.... **I admit that**.
Anxiety didn't beat me...**I am working on it**

Bradley Allan

Printed in Great Britain
by Amazon